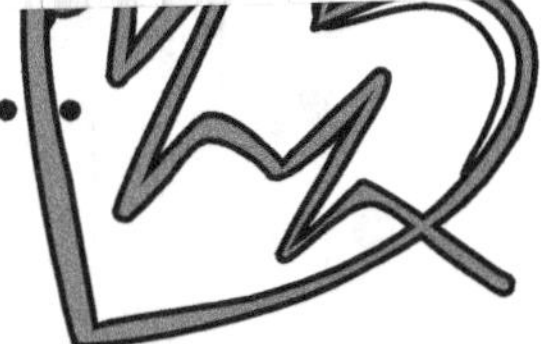

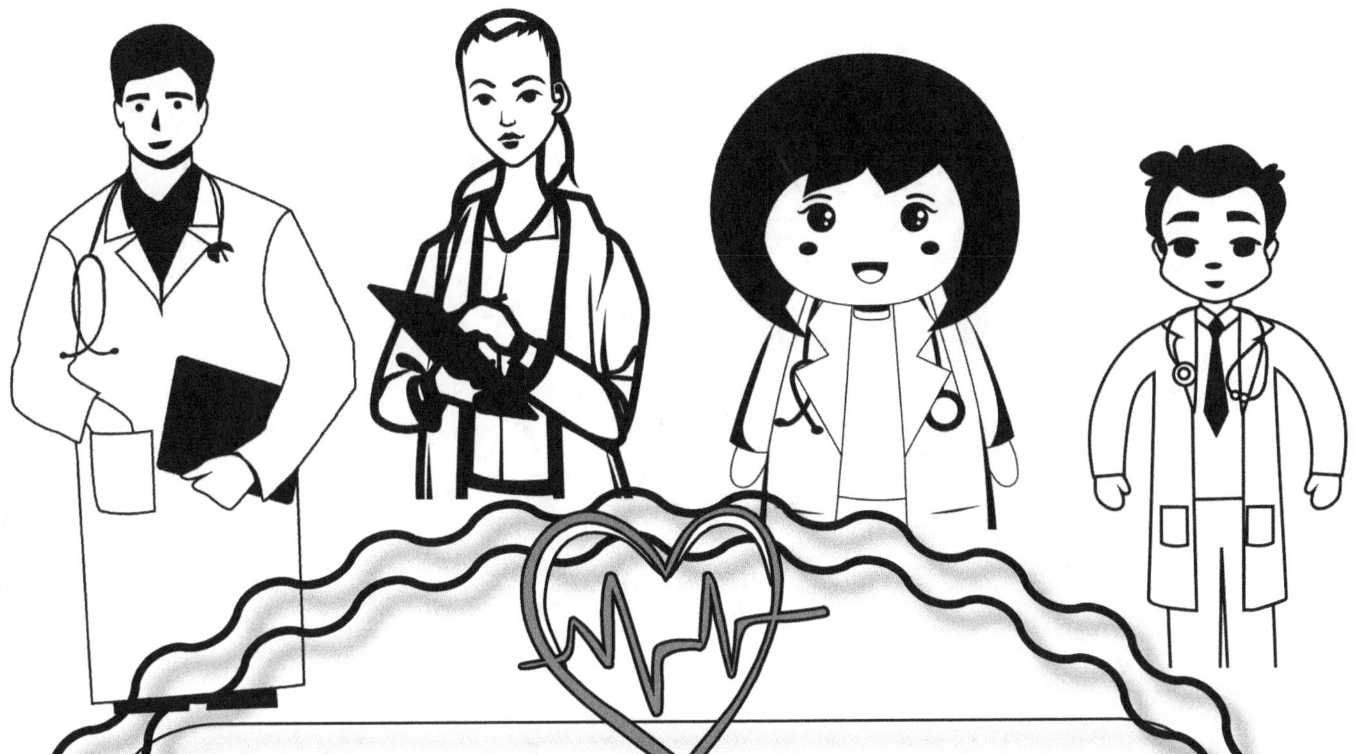

Simoun Chif

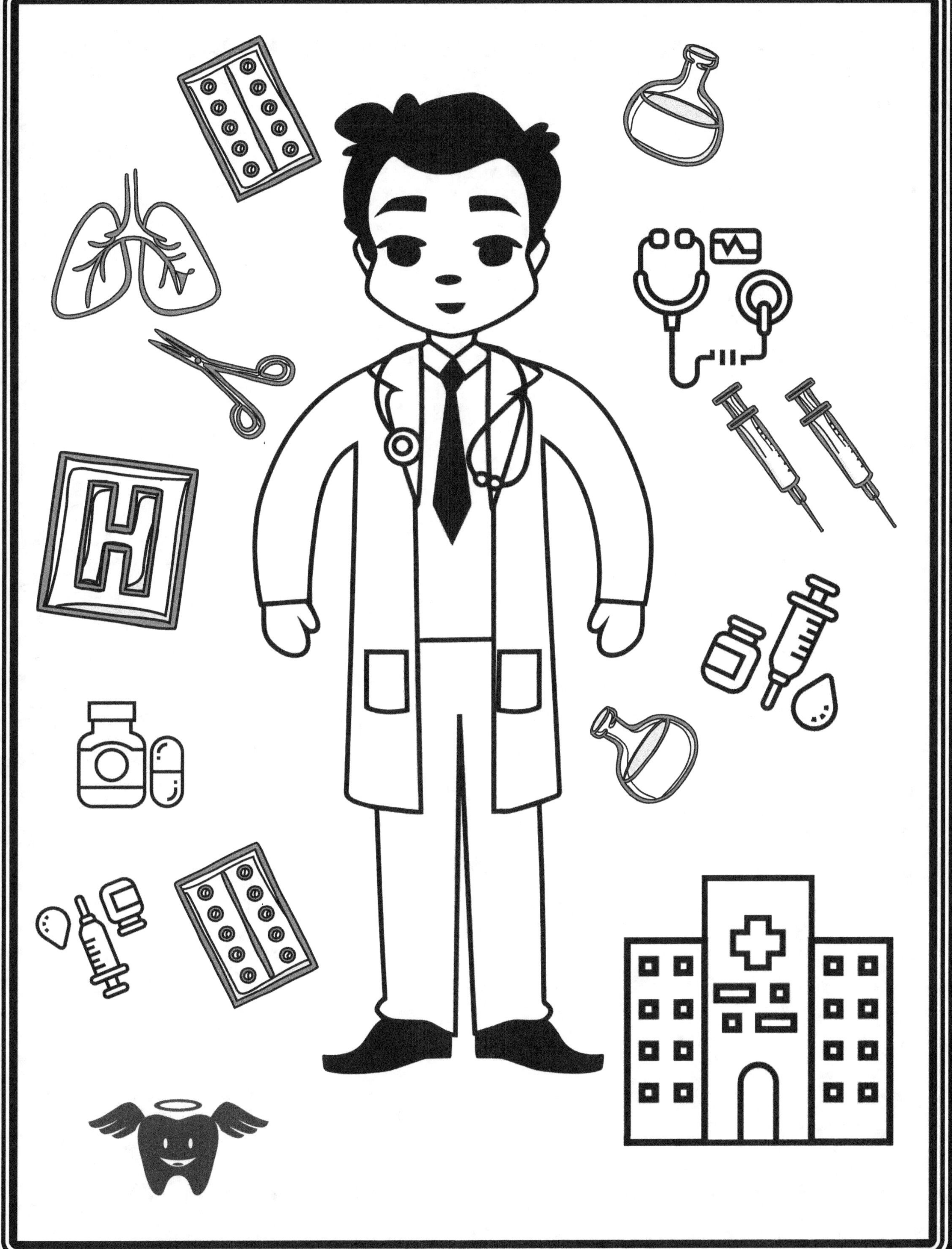

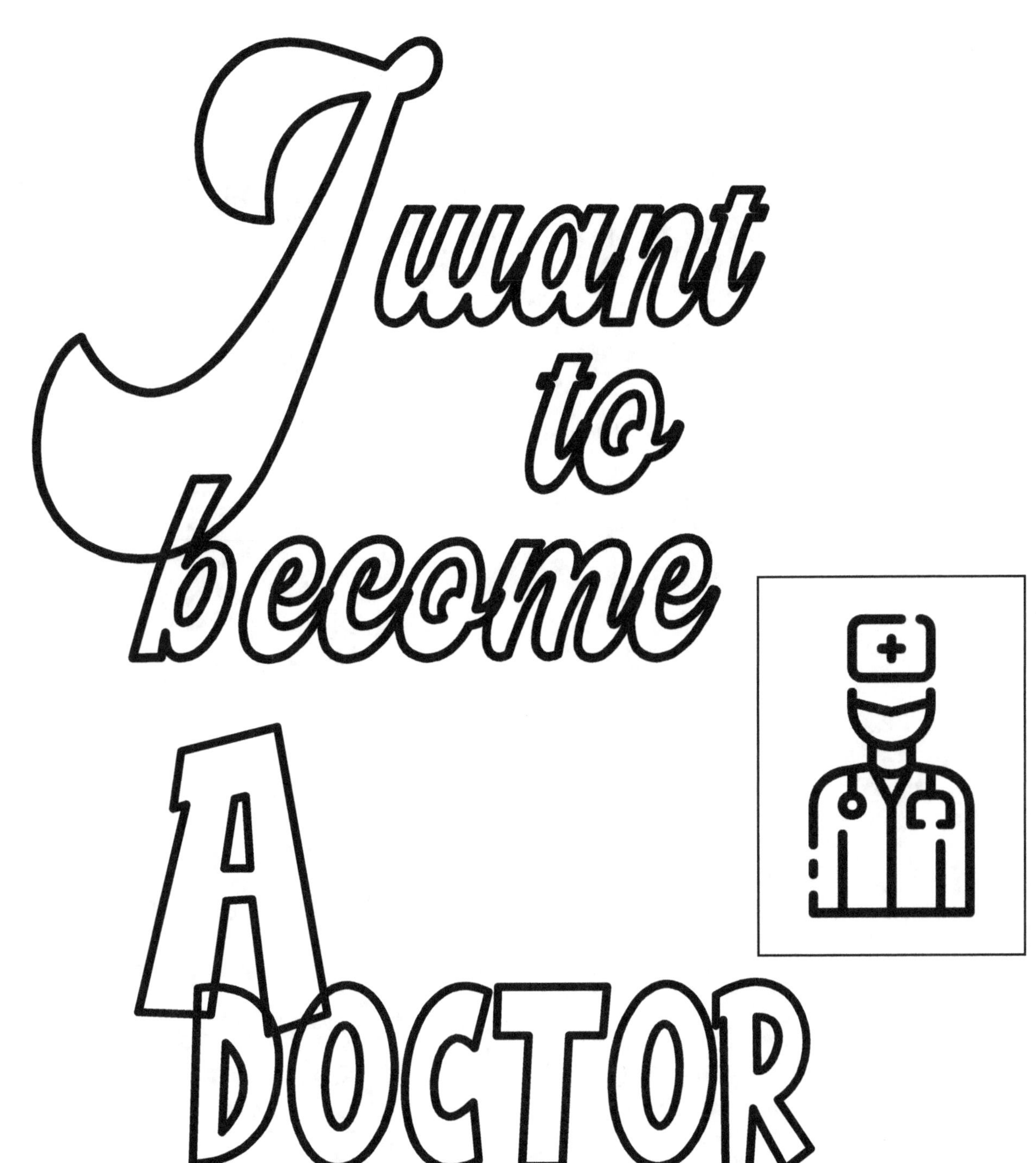

I want
to
become
A
DOCTOR

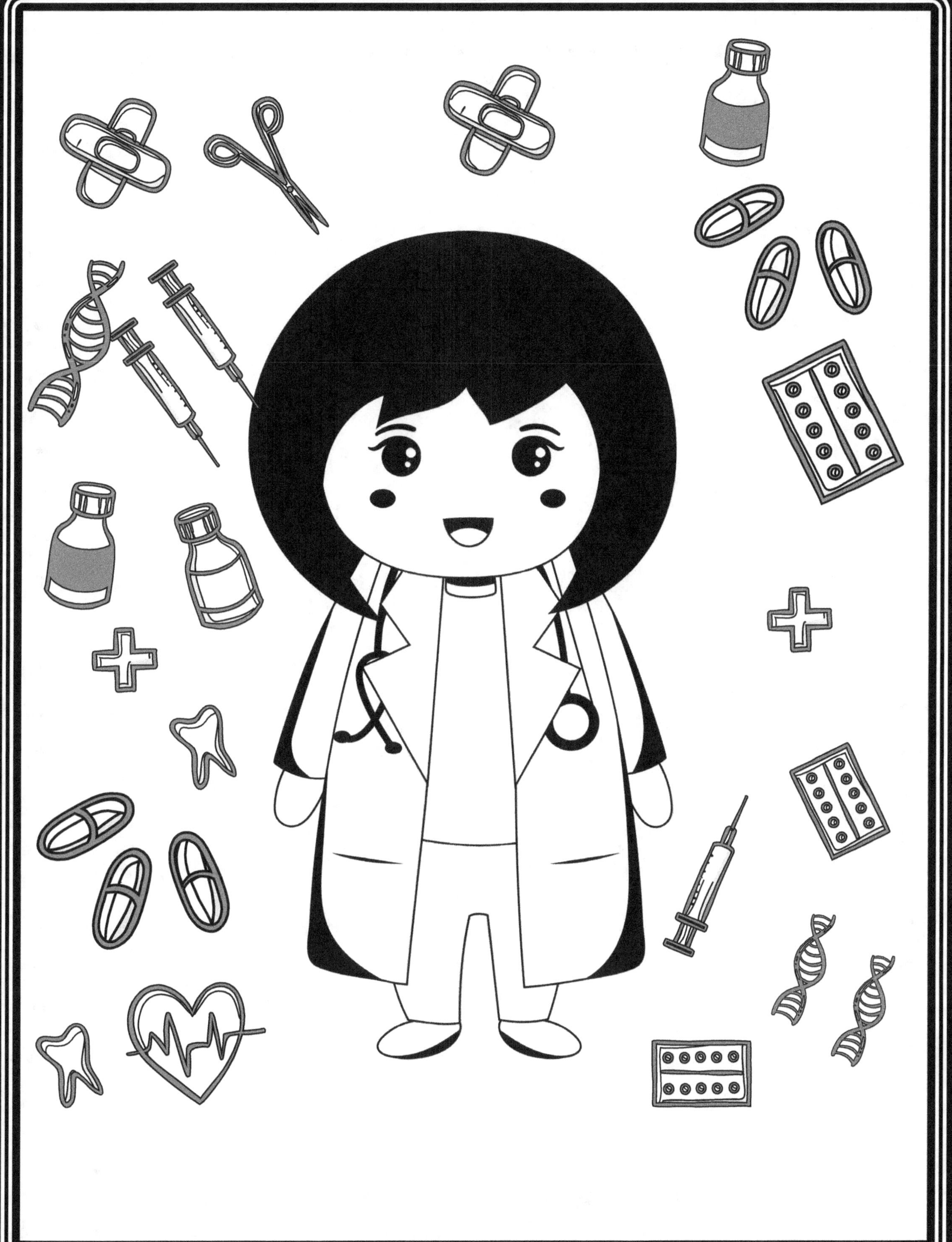

trist Me

I'm

the doctor

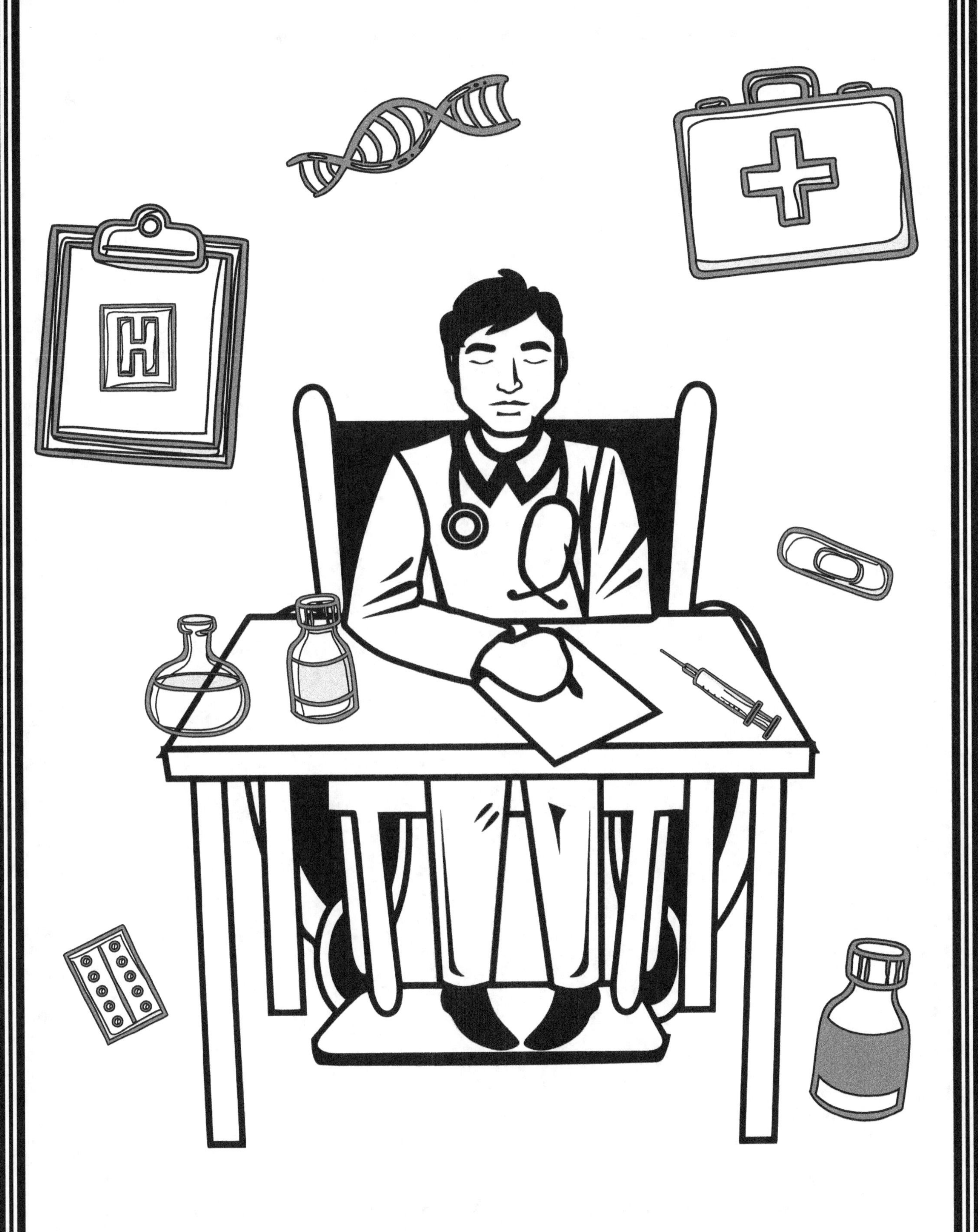

The best
doctor
gives
the
least
medicines.

THANKFUL FOR OUR

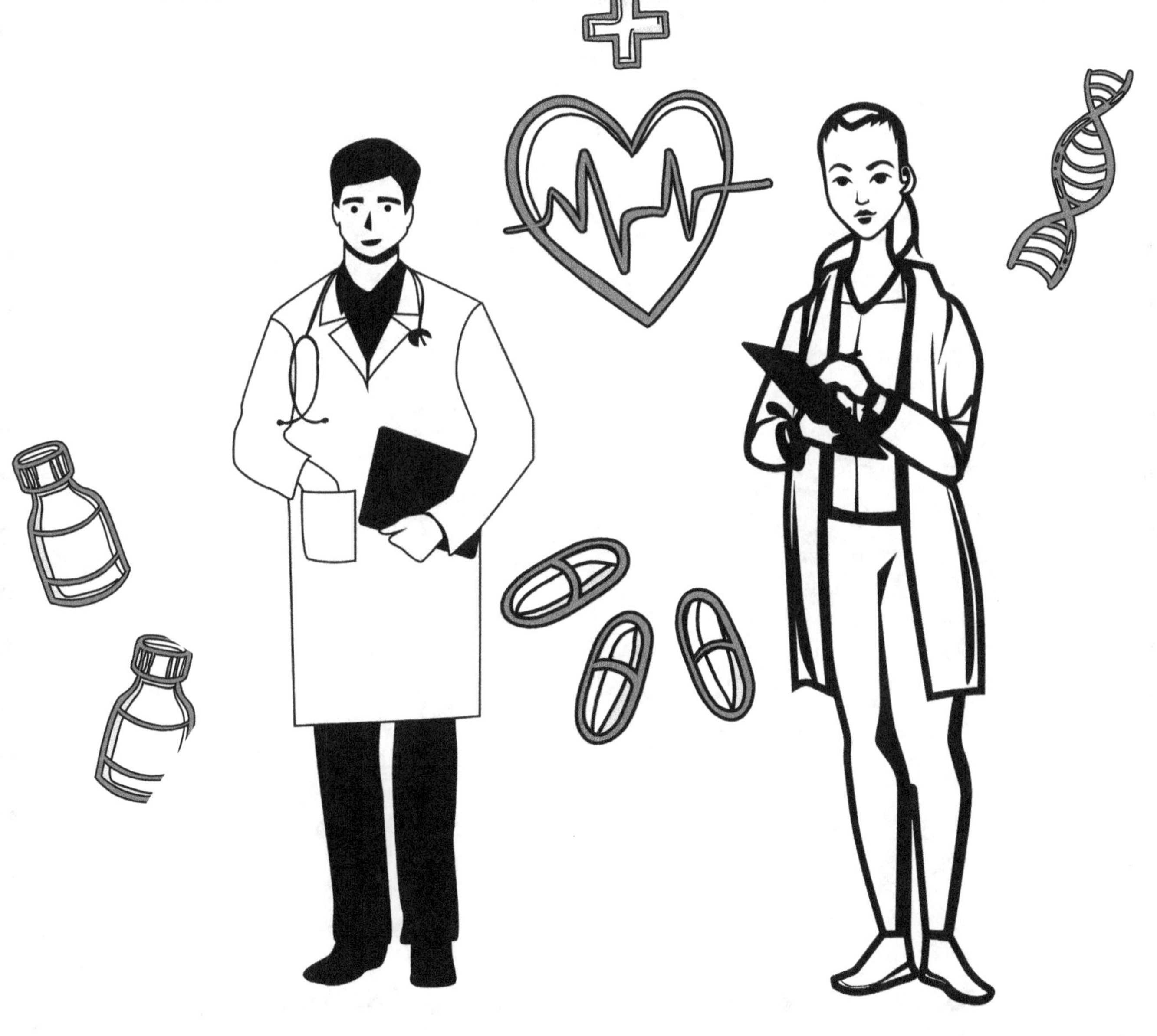

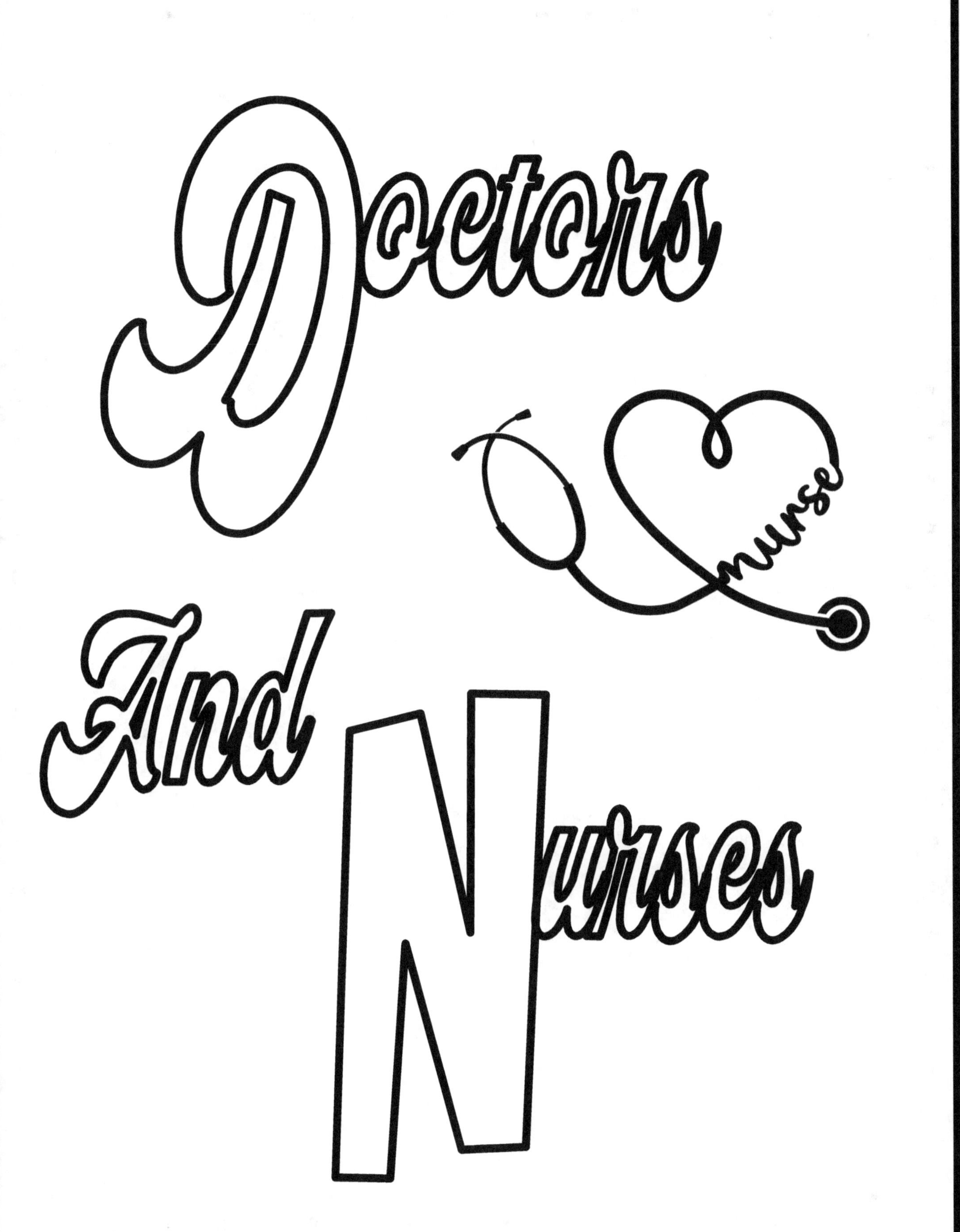

Doctors
And
Nurses
nurse

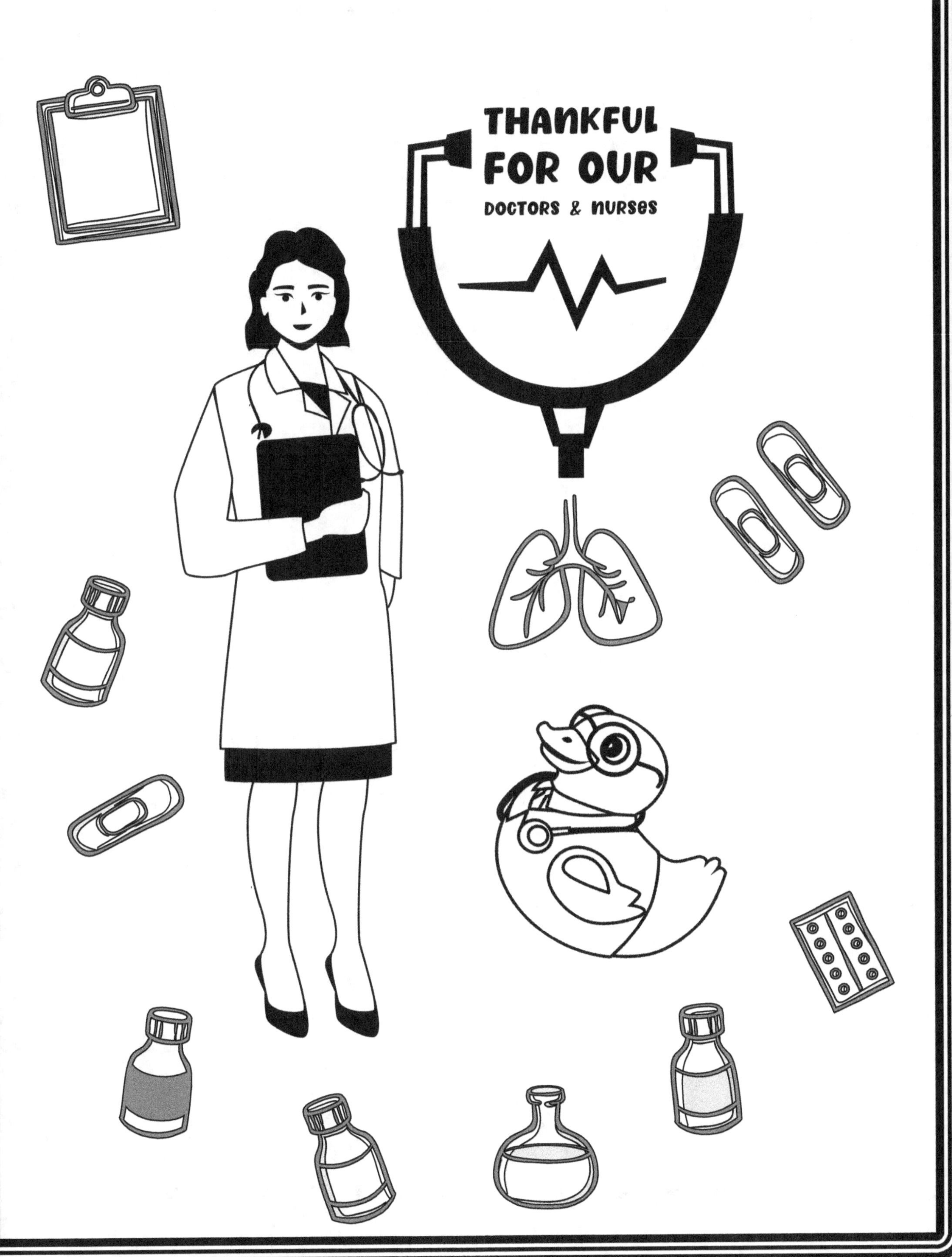

THANKFUL
FOR OUR
DOCTORS & NURSES

Complete :

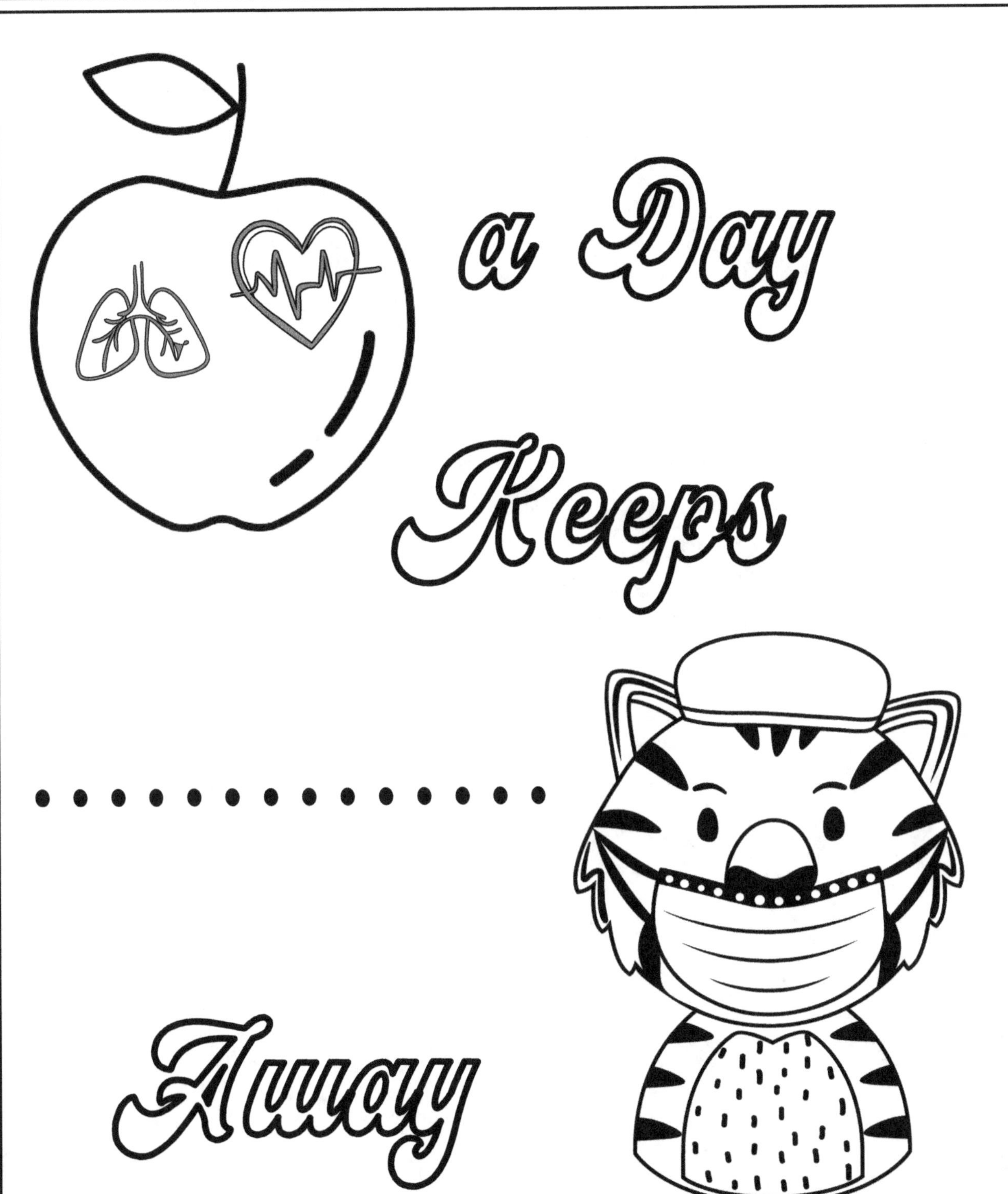

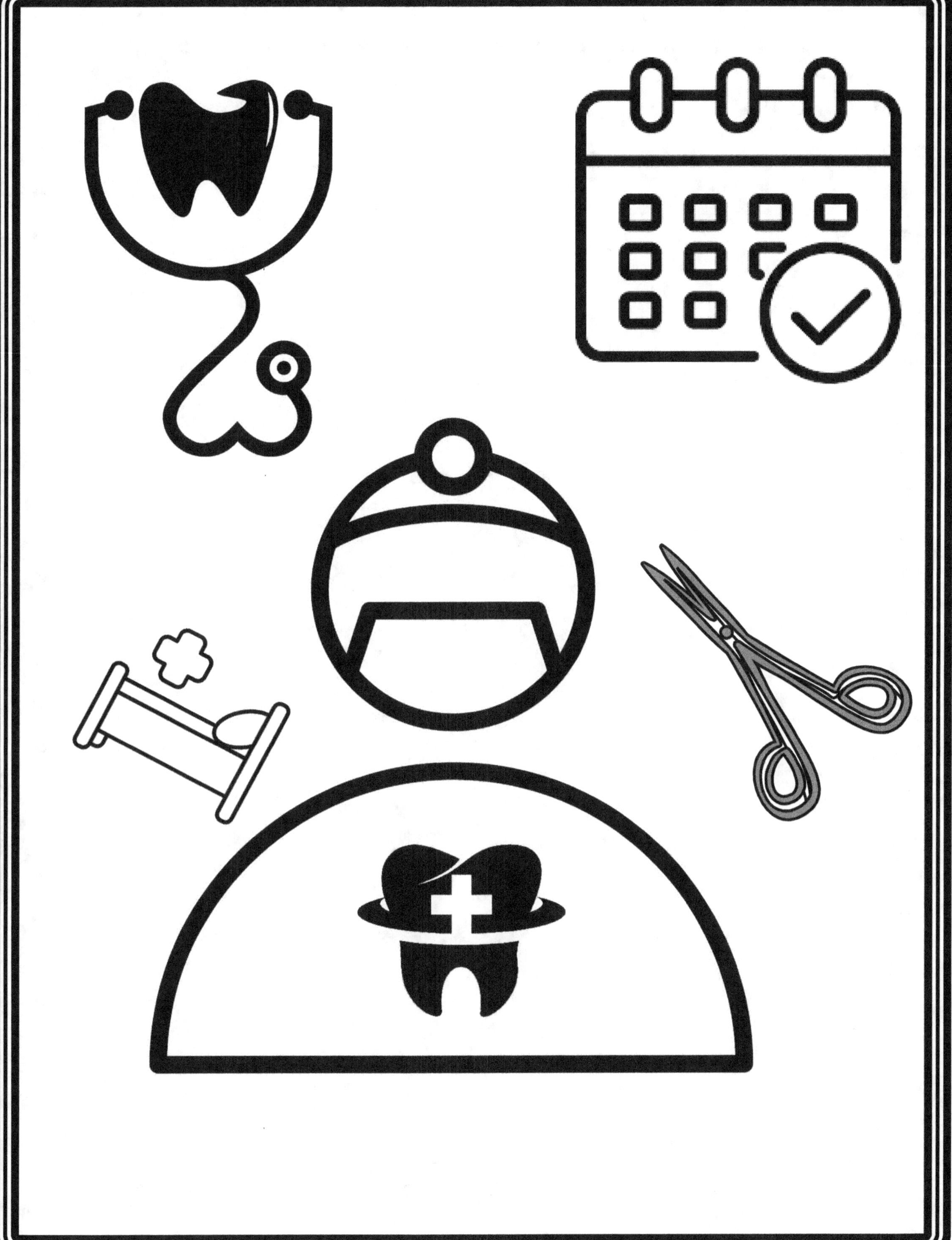

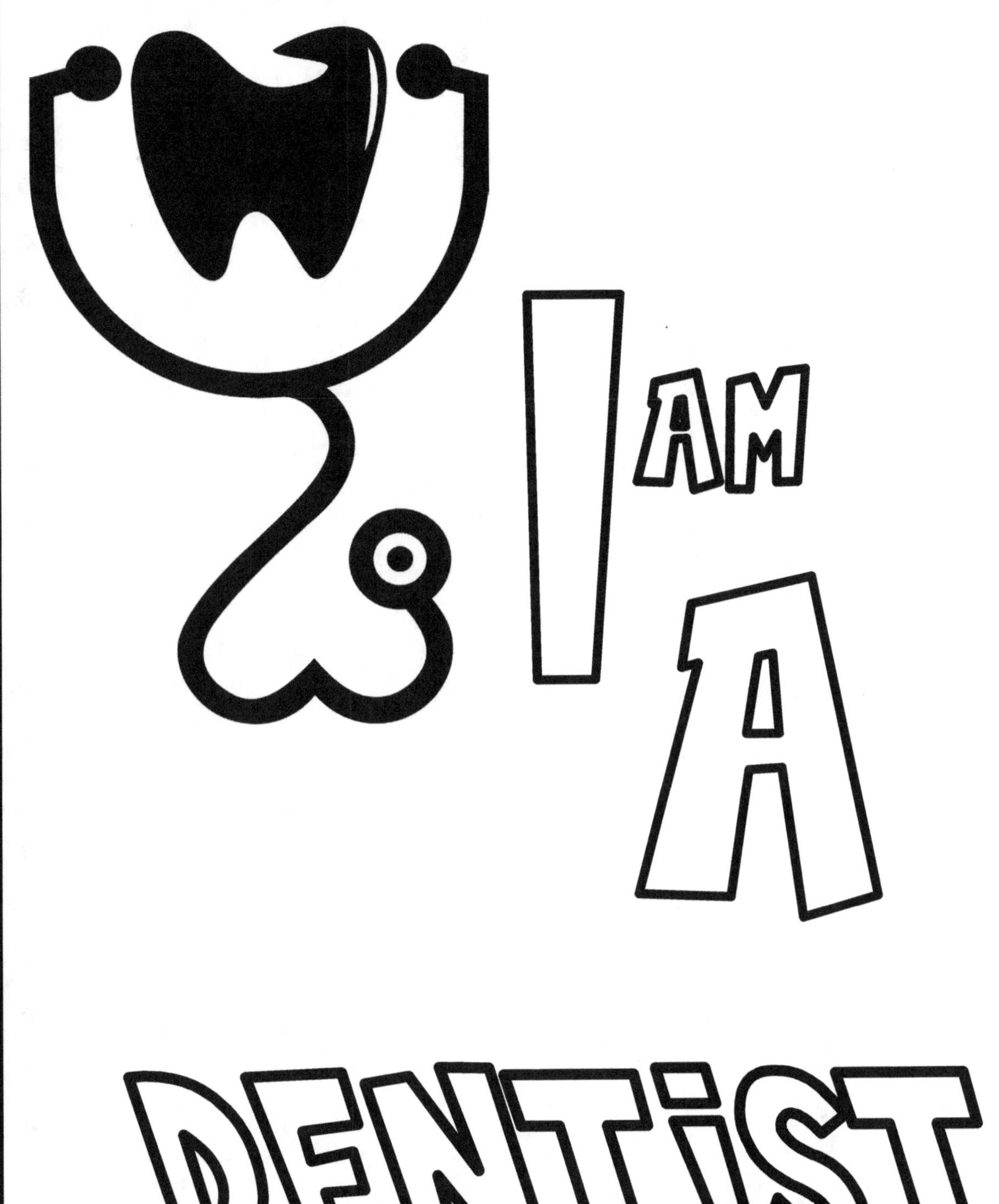

I AM A
DENTIST

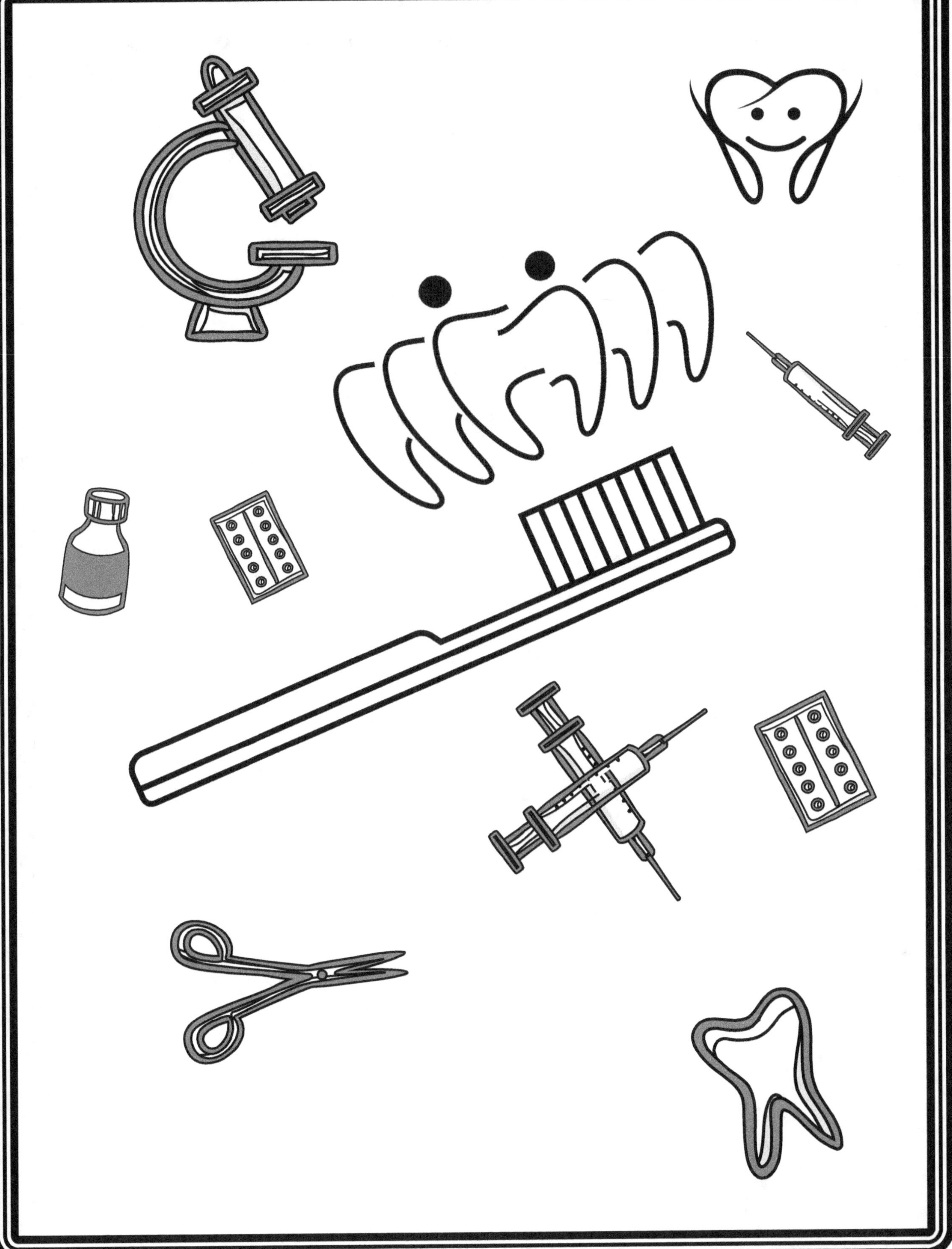

I BRUSH MY TEETH TWICE A DAY

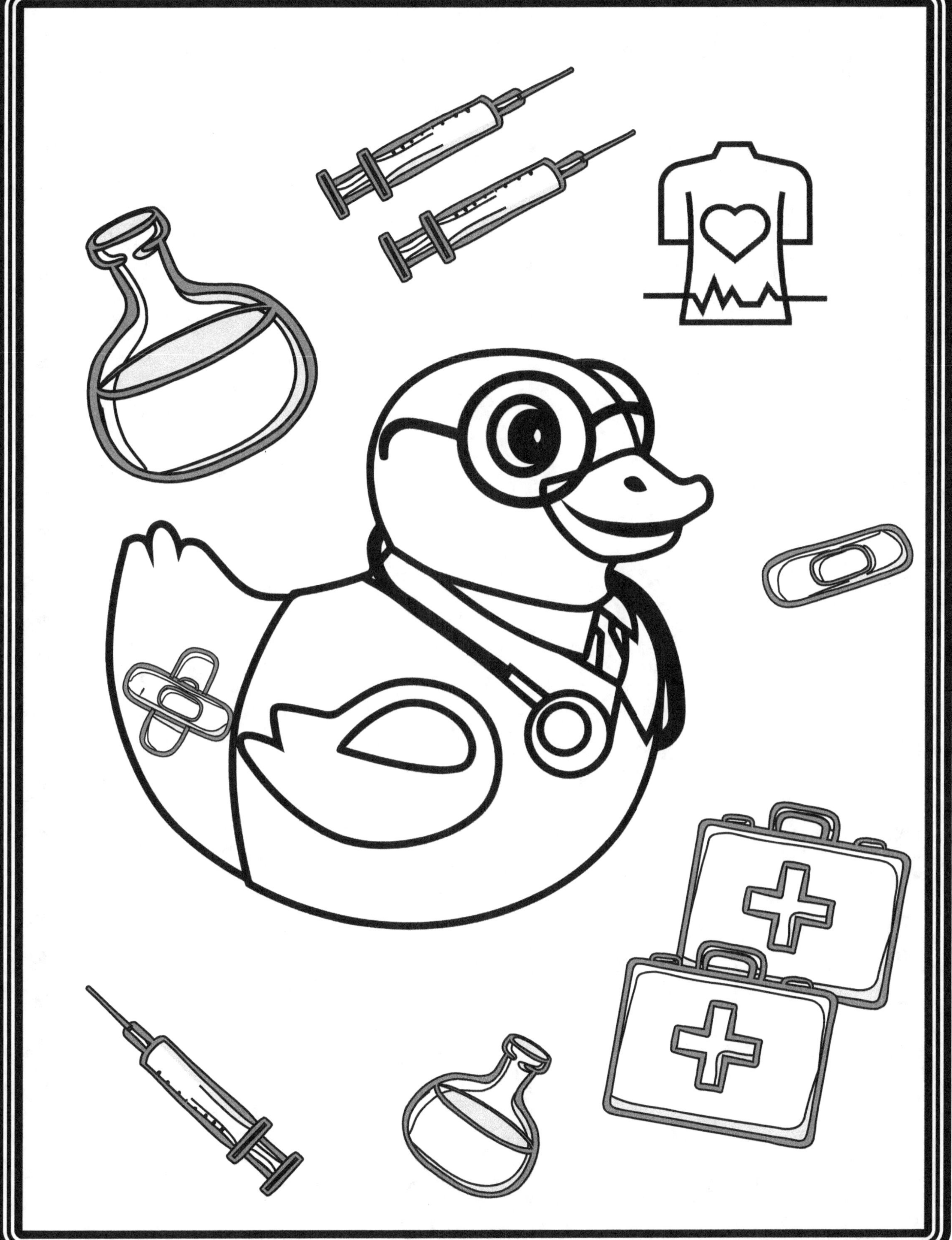

WHITENESS
OF MY
TEETH IS
MY SMILE

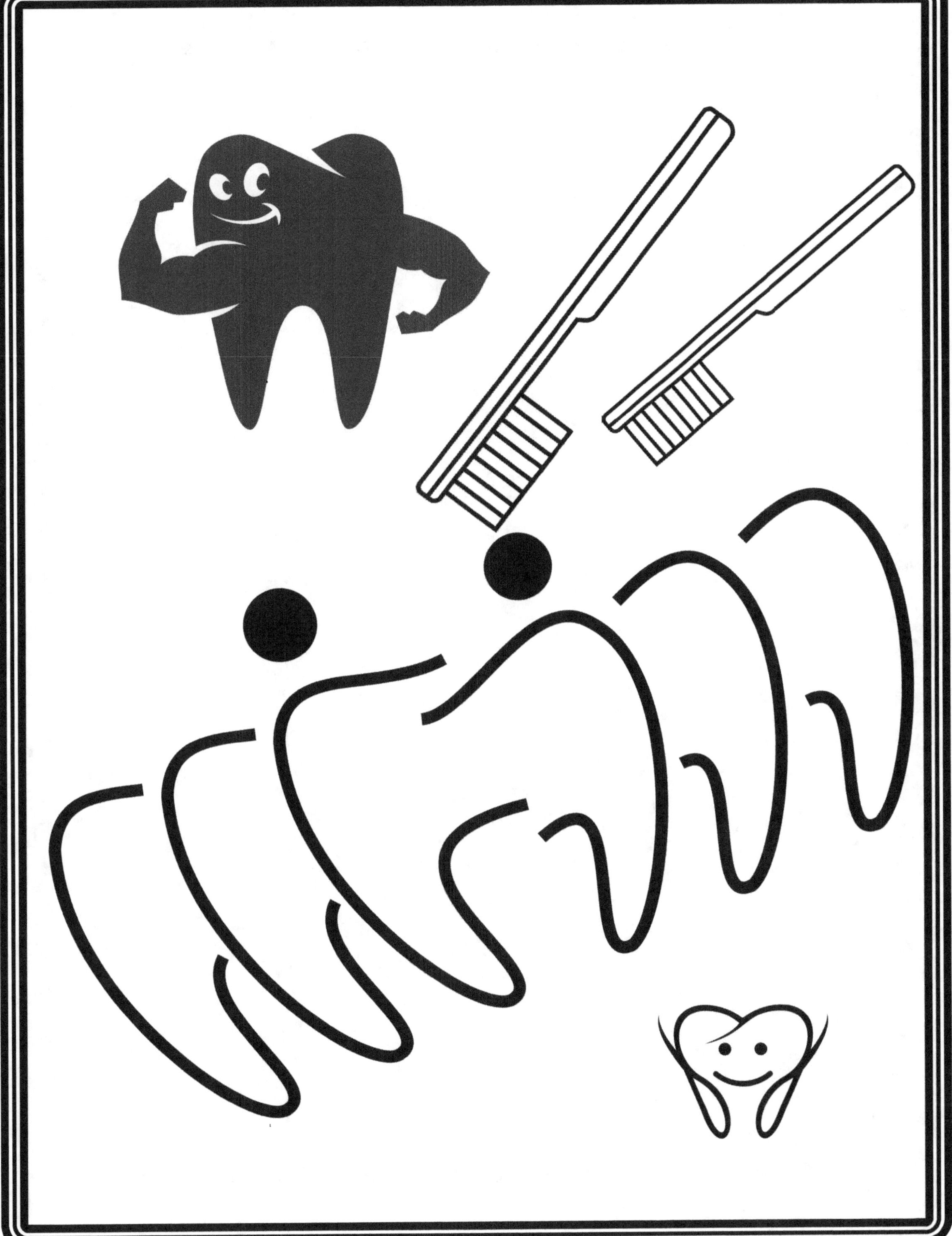

Don't Forget

Brush Your Teeth Every Day

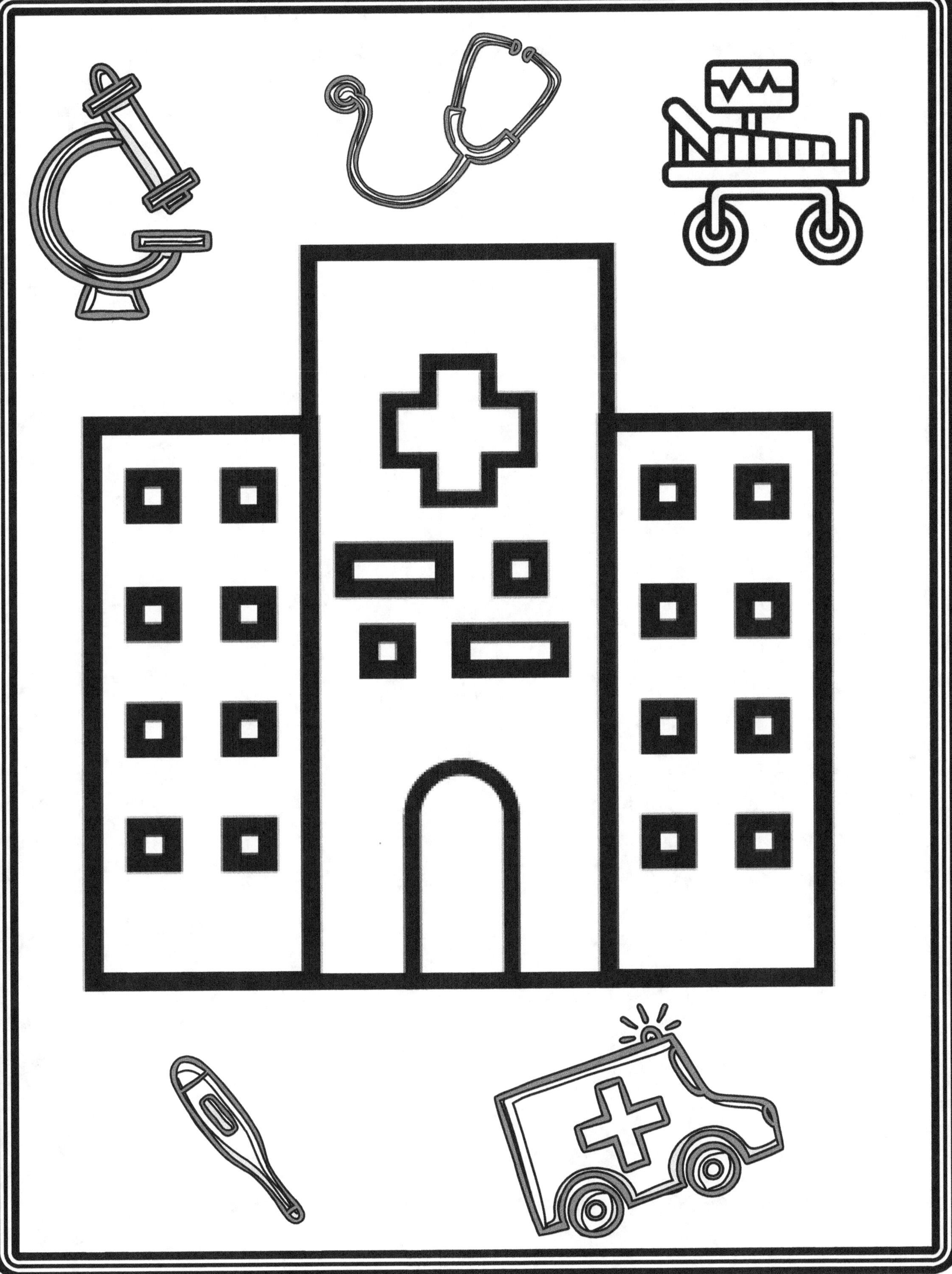

The hospital is A HEALTH INSTITUTION

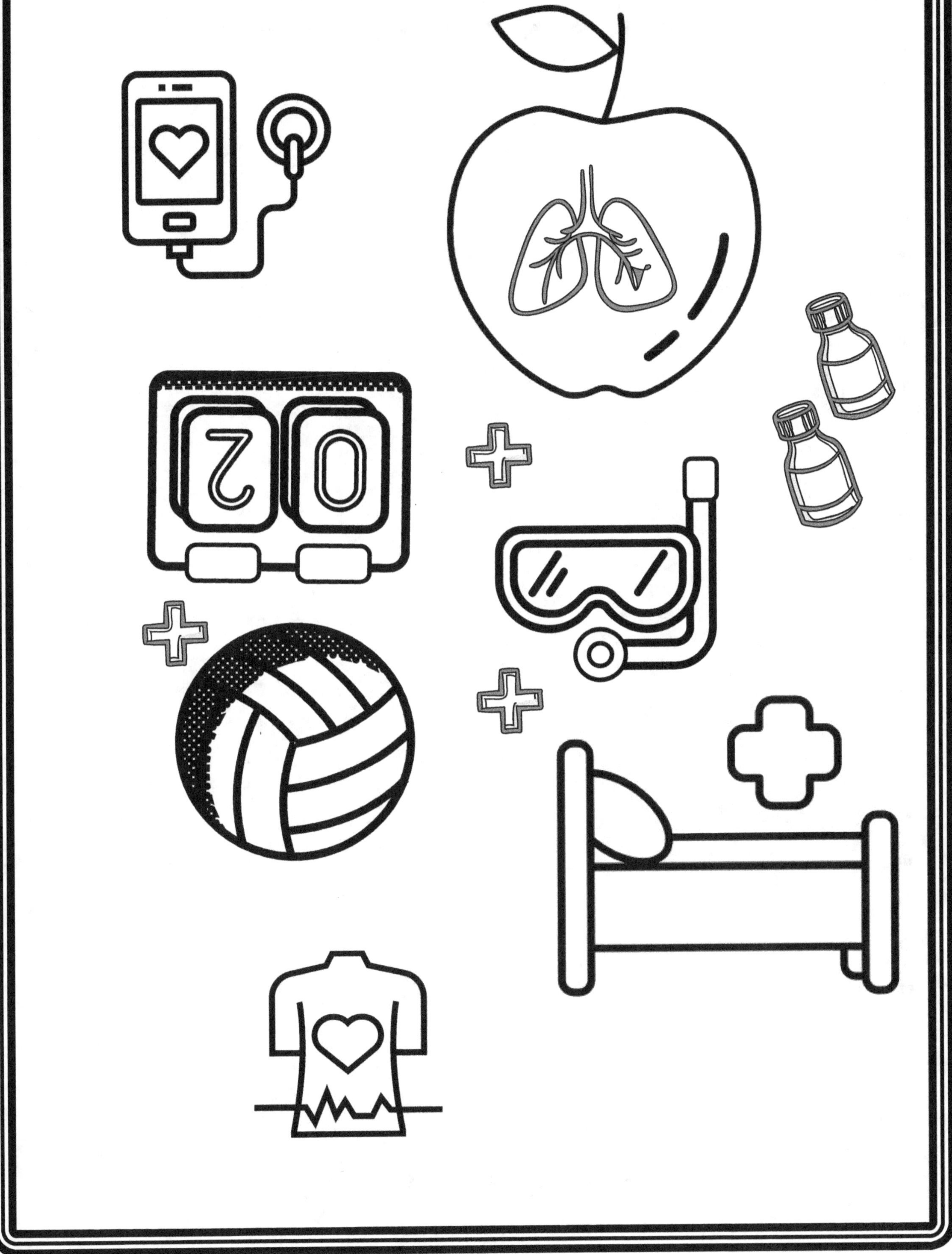

Eating

+

Sports

+

Sleep

=

a great Doctor

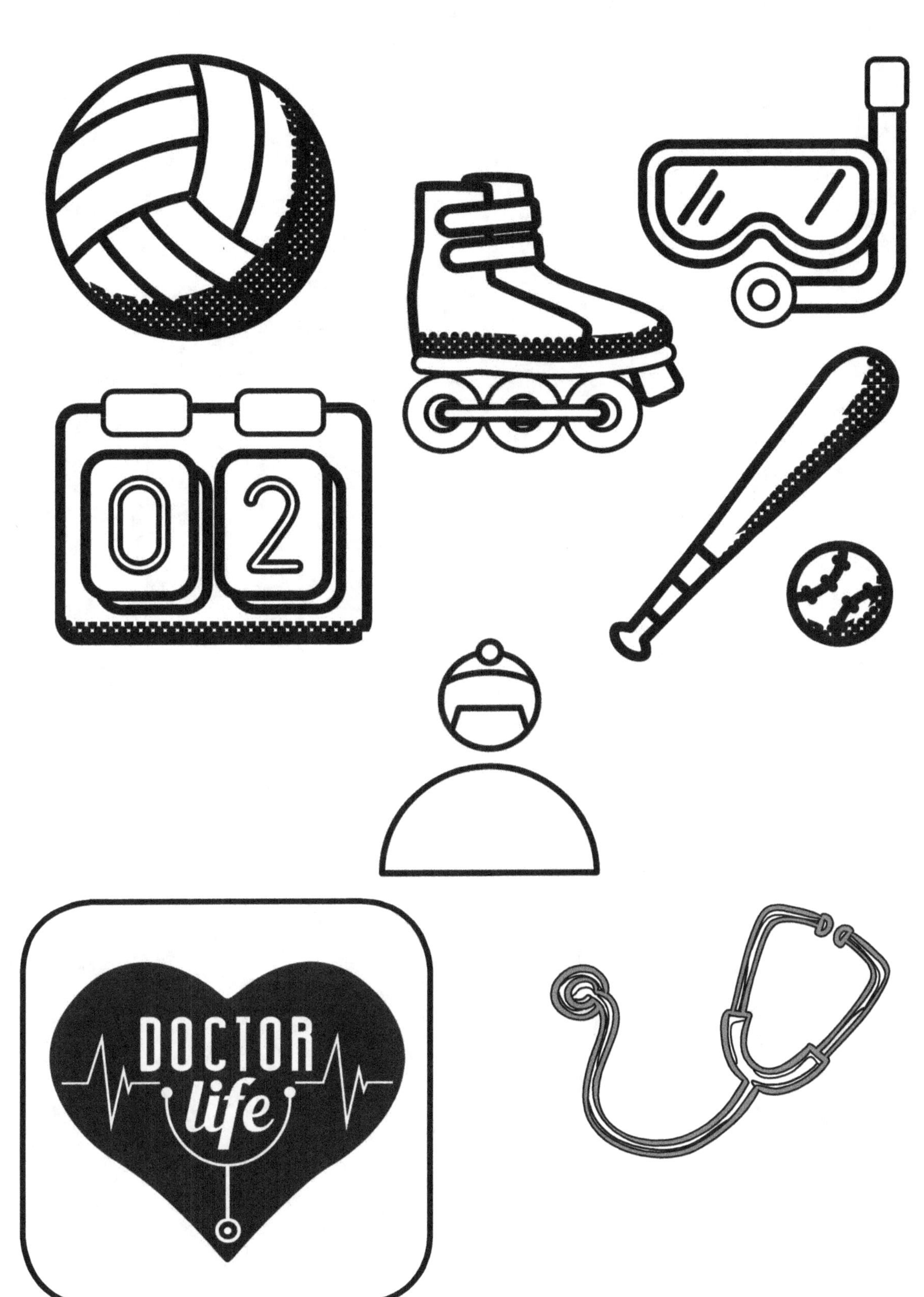

02
DOCTOR
life

I like sports and exercises